HEALTHY LIFESTYLE AGAINST HIGH BLOOD PRESSURE

How To Control Prevent And Reverse Hypertension

A nutritional and mindset approach

1st. Edition

Amie Armstrong

Disclaimer Notice:

Please note the information contained within this document is for educational and entertainment purposes only. Every attempt has been made to provide accurate, up to date and complete, reliable information. No warranties of any kind are expressed or implied. Readers acknowledge that the author is not engaging in the rendering of legal, financial, medical or professional advice. The content of this book has been derived from various sources. Please consult a licensed professional before attempting any techniques outlined in this book.

By reading this document, the reader agrees that under no circumstances is the author responsible for any losses, direct or indirect, which are incurred as a result of the use of information contained within this document, including, but not limited to, —errors, omissions, or inaccuracies.

Contents

INTRODUCTION

Blood is the fluid that circulates through the heart and blood vessels, supplying oxygen and nutritive materials to all parts of the body and carrying off waste products. Physiology of the blood cells Blood is composed of the following parts:- Red blood cells with their haemaeglobin; White blood cells, and Tiny little bodies much smaller than the red cells, which are called platelets

Hypertension is derived from two root words; Hyper meaning High and Tension meaning Pressure. Hypertension simply means high blood pressure. Pressure is the force generated when the heart contracts and pump blood through the blood vessels that conduct the blood to various parts of the blood.

Although hypertension does not mean or result from excessive emotional tension, but evidence shows that stress and emotional tension do cause increase in blood pressure, and if continuous, could be sustained.

High blood pressure is therefore generally defined as a blood pressure exceeding 140/90mmHg confirmed on multiple occasions. The top number (140) is called the SYSTOLIC PRESSURE, and it represents the pressure in the blood vessels (arteries) as the heart contracts and pump blood into circulation. The bottom number (90) is called DIASTOLIC PRESSURE, and it represents the pressure in the blood vessels as the heart relaxes after contraction. These figures measured in millimeters of Mercury (mmHg) reflect the highest and lowest pressures the heart and blood vessels are exposed to during circulation. The generally accepted normal value for blood pressure is 120/80mmHg. Above this value but less than 140/90mmHg is not considered to be hypertensive yet but signals danger, it is therefore called High normal.

An elevation of the blood pressure (Hypertension) increases the risk of developing Heart (Cardiac) diseases such as Heart Failure and Heart attack, Kidney diseases, Vascular diseases like athelosclerosis (hardening and narrowing of blood vessels), Eye damage and Stroke (brain damage).

These complications called End organ damage arise as a result of long standing (chronic) hypertension. But victims of hypertension are not aware, at an early stage, that they have the disease, until these complications start appearing. This is because hypertension shows virtually no signs/symptoms at the early stage. For this reason, it is generally referred to as the 'Silent Killer'.

CHAPTER 1- THE SILENT KILLER

High blood pressure, or hypertension, is a chronic medical condition where the arterial pressure of the blood is elevated. High blood pressure is a risk factor for heart attack, heart failure, stroke, and arterial aneurysm. Hypertension is also one of the leading causes of chronic kidney failure. The symptoms of elevated blood stress include headache, drowsiness, confusion, and nausea. Vision disorders such as blurred vision, color blindness, and vision loss can also develop because of high blood strain.

Lifestyle changes are recommended to prevent elevated blood pressure, and also to treat it before the initiation of prescription drug therapy. Recommended lifestyle changes include weight loss and regular aerobic exercise to improve blood flow and reduce the resting heart rate. Reducing salt and sugar in the diet is also an effective measure. Increasing potassium in one's diet can offset the effects of salt, or sodium. It is also beneficial to have a diet rich in fruits and vegetables, and to consume low-fat or fat-free dairy products. Discontinuing tobacco use and limiting alcohol consumption to less than two drinks per day can reduce blood strain, as well. Reducing stress is another effective way to lower blood pressure. Relaxation techniques and cognitive therapy can reduce negative stress responses in the body. Other stress reduction techniques include avoiding over-illumination and high sound levels.

Doctors usually diagnose a patient with hypertension on the basis of persistently high blood stress. This typically requires three measurements during separate visits to a doctor's office at least one week apart. However, if a patient's blood pressure is extremely high, or if symptoms of organ damage are evident, then diagnosis and treatments may be given immediately. Following diagnosis, the initial line of treatment for high blood strain is usually the same as the lifestyle changes used as preventative measures. In addition to recommended lifestyle changes, doctors may prescribe several different classes of medications, collectively known as antihypertensive drugs. Doctors often combine multiple drugs to achieve the target blood pressure level for a patient.

High blood pressure is the most important risk factor for death in developed countries in the world. Professional health care is an important part of treating elevated blood pressure. While people with high blood stress often display symptoms, many people have mild to moderate hypertension without showing any signs. It is important to see a doctor to determine if you have or are at risk of developing high blood pressure.

Healthy lifestyle is the best treatment for high blood pressure

Effective High Blood Pressure Treatments

If you have high blood pressure, you will have to take action to treat it. If ignored, hypertension can lead to very serious health problems including stroke, heart disease and kidney failure. So what high blood pressure treatments are the most effective? Find out what works best to keep blood pressure under control.

No drug can ever help you to win a battle against high blood pressure for good. The best they can do is to give a temporarily relief. However, by changing your lifestyle habits you can keep your blood pressure under control.

There are 3 major aspects of your life that affect blood pressure

- Exercise

- Diet

- Stress management

Making your heart beating slightly faster than normal from time to time is very important. This doesn't mean you will have to go the gym every day. Many everyday things count as exercise - house chores, gardening, walking your dog or playing active games with your children are good examples. Walking is the best exercise for high blood pressure, even 15 minutes a day will do wonder. Most important you should do some exercise every day.

Another essential thing you will have to evaluate is your diet. Do you like souses, pickles and pre-cooked meals? Then you will have to cut it down, because all of the above are extremely high in sodium and sodium affects blood pressure very badly. Add more veggies and fruits to your diet, remove your salt shaker from the table and you will feel much better as your blood pressure lowers.

Every time you stress out, your blood pressure jumps up. And if stress is a permanent part of your life it can constantly keep your readings high. Don't ignore stress; there are many effective ways to deal with it. For example, you can enroll in a stress relief class or take a yoga or Tai Chi class. Try to find time to do things that you enjoy.

High blood pressure medication

When it comes to high blood pressure drugs, you should never get one without consulting a doctor. If a particular medicine works well for your friend it doesn't mean it will suit you. Most high blood pressure drugs are prescription drugs, so the only way to get them is to visit your physician first and ask for prescription.

Medication used to control high blood pressure includes:

- ACE inhibitors

- Calcium channel blockers

- Beta-blockers

- Angiotensin-receptor blockers (ARBs)

- Alpha-blockers

- Diuretics

In the past a lot of high blood pressure medications were unsafe and had side effects. Luckily they improved in recent years, so modern drugs that help to lower your blood pressure are more effective and safe.

Alternative high blood pressure treatments

If you don't trust conventional drugs and prefer alternative medicine, there are several treatments that can help to lower blood pressure.

Natural herbs for high blood pressure are very popular. Most effective are Hawthorn and Ginkgo Biloba. Several studies have shown that garlic also helps with hypertension control. Garlic thins the blood (reduces its ability to clot). Garlic supplements work just as well as fresh garlic.

Among the alternative therapies, most common are acupuncture and magnetic high blood pressure therapy.

Acupuncture relaxes your body and releases some of the strain on the heart. There is no hard scientific proof that acupunctures works, but many people who tried it, swear that it helped to decrease their blood pressure.

Treatment with magnets can also help. Copper and iron bracelets reduce the effects of blood pressure, but scientists don't know how and why. However, this treatment is painless and safe, so it is worth the try.

There are many ways to treat high blood pressure. You should never ignore it, because this condition doesn't just go away unless you do something to control it.

CHAPTER 2- How TO CONTROL HYPERTENSION

Hypnotherapy to Reduce Blood Pressure

If you have blood pressure problems then you may need to take action to help control hypertension. Hypertension, when left unchecked can lead to all sorts of health care problems. You need to get the support it will take to get your blood pressure under control ꞏuickly. The good news is that there is more than one thing that helps lower hypertension and bring your pressure under control. Not all of these things are medicinal or chemical in nature.

Stress and Hypertension

If you really want to do something that will help control hypertension then you want to reduce the amount of stress and anxiety in your daily routine. There are believed to be two of the primary culprits for high blood pressure and the various associated problems.

Stress and anxiety can make a bad situation worse, very quickly when it comes to high blood pressure and your health.

This is a condition that you do not want to gamble with. The consequences of doing so may be much more costly than you anticipate. Make sure that you are putting your health ahead of everything else and getting the help control to hypertension you need. Don't become another statistic of poor health care for hypertension and blood pressure related problems- learn all you can to help control hypertension today and rid your life of this albatross.

Relaxation for Hypertension

Learning deep relaxation exercises, taking up a low stress hobby, getting in a little bit of low impact exercise, or even taking up yoga can greatly reduce the amount of stress and anxiety that you carry around with you. This in effect will also lower the amount of hypertension you experience. The point is to make a plan to incorporate a little relaxation into your life. You deserve it after all and it can save your life if you let it. It will also make you a little bit easier to live with.

Hypnotherapy for Hypertension

One way, that is receiving more and more acclaim to treat hypertension and high blood pressure is with the use of hypnotherapy or NLP (neuro-linguistic programming). An NLP therapist with your best interest in mind will require that you receive a physicians care along with your hypnotherapy if you've been diagnosed as having high blood pressure. This will ensure that you are getting the best possible care and that you will truly be able to help control hypertension from the very beginning.

Neuro-linguistic treatment programs work to help control hypertension because they teach your mind to get the upper hand. When you put your mind in charge, as it should be, you will receive much better results for your efforts at lowering your blood pressure. This works because NLP can be used to program your body to be balanced in combination with hypnosis for hypertension that is mean to help you relax, lower your stress level, and get the sleep you need to succeed.

CHAPTER 3- PREVENTING FROM KILLER

You can help prevent high blood pressure by having a healthy lifestyle. This means

Eating a healthy diet. To help manage your blood pressure, you should limit the amount of sodium (salt) that you eat, and increase the amount of potassium in your diet. It is also important to eat foods that are lower in fat, as well as plenty of fruits, vegetables, and whole grains. The DASH diet is an example of an eating plan that can help you to lower your blood pressure.

Getting regular exercise. Exercise can help you maintain a healthy weight and lower your blood pressure. You should try to get moderate-intensity aerobic exercise at least 2 and a half hours per week, or vigorous-intensity aerobic exercise for 1 hour and 15 minutes per week. Aerobic exercise, such as brisk walking, is any exercise in which your heart beats harder and you use more oxygen than usual.

Being at a healthy weight. Being overweight or having obesity increases your risk for high blood pressure.

Maintaining a healthy weight can help you control high blood pressure and reduce your risk for other health problems.

Limiting alcohol. Drinking too much alcohol can raise your blood pressure. It also adds extra calories, which may cause weight gain. Men should have no more than two drinks per day, and women only one.

Not smoking. Cigarette smoking raises your blood pressure and puts you at higher risk for heart attack and stroke. If you do not smoke, do not start. If you do smoke, talk to your health care provider for help in finding the best way for you to ▢uit.

Managing stress. Learning how to relax and manage stress can improve your emotional and physical health and lower high blood pressure. Stress management techniques include exercising, listening to music, focusing on something calm or peaceful, and meditating.

Blood pressure is the force of your blood pushing against the walls of your arteries. Each time your heart beats, it pumps blood into the arteries. Your blood pressure is highest when your heart beats, pumping the blood. This is called systolic pressure. When your heart is at rest, between beats, your blood pressure falls. This is called diastolic pressure.

Your blood pressure reading uses these two numbers. Usually the systolic number comes before or above the diastolic number.

How do I know if my blood pressure is high?

High blood pressure usually has no symptoms. So the only way to find out if you have high blood pressure is to get regular blood pressure checks from your health care provider. Your provider will use a gauge, a stethoscope or electronic sensor, and a blood pressure cuff. For most adults, blood pressure readings will be in one of four categories:

Normal blood pressure means

Your systolic pressure is less than 120 AND

Your diastolic pressure is less than 80

Prehypertension means

Your systolic pressure is between 120-139 OR

Your diastolic pressure is between 80-89

Stage 1 high blood pressure means

Your systolic pressure is between 140-159 OR

Your diastolic pressure is between 90-99

Stage 2 high blood pressure means

Your systolic pressure is 160 or higher OR

Your diastolic pressure is 100 or higher

For children and teens, the health care provider compares the blood pressure reading to what is normal for other kids who are the same age, height, and gender.

People with diabetes or chronic kidney disease should keep their blood pressure below 130/80.

Why do I need to worry about prehypertension and high blood pressure?

Prehypertension means you're likely to end up with high blood pressure, unless you take steps to prevent it.

When your blood pressure stays high over time, it causes the heart to pump harder and work overtime, possibly leading to serious health problems such as heart attack, stroke, heart failure, and kidney failure.

What are the different types of high blood pressure?

There are two main types of high blood pressure: primary and secondary high blood pressure.

Primary, or essential, high blood pressure is the most common type of high blood pressure. For most people who get this kind of blood pressure, it develops over time as you get older.

Secondary high blood pressure is caused by another medical condition or use of certain medicines. It usually gets better after you treat the cause or stop taking the medicines that are causing it.

Who is at risk for high blood pressure?

Anyone can develop high blood pressure, but there are certain factors that can increase your risk:

Age - Blood pressure tends to rise with age

Race/Ethnicity - High blood pressure is more common in African American adults

Weight - People who are overweight or have obesity are more likely to develop prehypertension or high blood pressure

Gender - Before age 55, men are more likely than women to develop high blood pressure. After age 55, women are more likely than men to develop it.

Lifestyle - Certain lifestyle habits can raise your risk for high blood pressure, such as eating too much sodium or not enough potassium, lack of exercise, drinking too much alcohol, and smoking.

Family history - A family history of high blood pressure raises the risk of developing prehypertension or high blood pressure

Changing lifestyle can also be necessary in conjunction with taking medication. In other cases, it may be possible to eliminate medication if the appropriate changes are made in lifestyle. With some people medication will be taken along with changing lifestyle until improvements are reached. But more and more sufferers are finding a new way to control their hypertension.

Sometimes making simple diet corrections may not make a big difference. Just reducing salt intake will be a noticeable improvement. Do not eliminate every favorite food; make better choices and control portion size. Be sure to get plenty of water daily to keep hydrated.

CHAPTER 4- REVERSES HYPERTENSION

Making lifestyle changes and high blood pressure

A main lifestyle changes you can make that will help to lower your blood pressure. Some of them will lower your blood pressure in a matter of weeks; others will take a little longer. The changes are listed below in order of speed of effect:

Cut down on salt. This means eating more natural foods and fewer processed ones and not adding any extra salt to foods or in anything you cook. Salt naturally raises your blood pressure, eating less will reduce this effect. Please see the salt information page on our main site.

Increase the amount of fresh fruit and vegetables you eat each day. Aim to eat at least five, or better still seven to nine portions a day. It's also best to eat a variety of different fruit and vegetables. Fruit and vegetables contain potassium that counters the effect of salt and helps to lower blood pressure. Please see the fruit and vegetables page on our main site.

Drink alcohol only in moderation. No more than 2-3 units per day for men and women. Drinking more than the recommended limits over a long period will slowly raise your blood pressure. Please see the alcohol page on our main site.

Increase your level of activity. Build in 30 minutes of moderate activity at least five times per week. Being active not only gives your heart a good work out, but it also helps your arteries to stay flexible and better able to cope with the demands of daily life. Please see the physical activity page on our main site.

Lose weight if you are overweight. Your doctor or nurse will be able to tell you your ideal weight. Excess weight puts extra strain on your heart and your arteries. Please see the managing your weight page on our main site.

The good news is that these changes really do work and will help to lower your blood pressure for life.

The more changes you make, the more benefit you will gain and the greater the effect is likely to be on lowering your blood pressure. In fact some people find that, by sticking to a healthy lifestyle, they don't need to take any medicines at all. For example, if you have a lot of weight to lose and are able to achieve this, you may find that you no longer need to take medicines.

Ways To Control Hypertension

Many conditions like stroke, heart attack, aneurysm, kidney failure and heart failure are the result of a chronic medical condition known as hypertension. Many ways to control hypertension is by simply making lifestyle changes. For others that suffer with high blood pressure, medication combined with lifestyle changes may be required to manage the condition.

When diagnosed, many anti hypertensive drugs are available for physicians to prescribe. There is evidence to support that these medications can lower blood pressure as much as 5 mmHg and can reduce the possibility of stroke by more than thirty percent. Medication can also reduce the chances for coronary artery disease, dementia, death and cardiovascular disease more than twenty percent.

Changing lifestyle can also be necessary in conjunction with taking medication. In other cases, it may be possible to eliminate medication if the appropriate changes are made in lifestyle. With some people medication will be taken along with changing lifestyle until improvements are reached. But more and more sufferers are finding a new way to control their hypertension.

Sometimes making simple diet corrections may not make a big difference. Just reducing salt intake will be a noticeable improvement. Do not eliminate every favorite food; make better choices and control portion size. Be sure to get plenty of water daily to keep hydrated.

Often people are predisposed to the condition, but finding ways to control hypertension is more than possible. Smoking needs to be the first habit eliminated if it is a problem. Add some routine exercise; make better diet choices and there is a possibility that the condition can be controlled without medication at some point. Recently many victims of HBP who have tried the above suggestions with no results have had great success with an all-natural supplement designed especially for hypertension sufferers.

How to Control Hypertension

Combating with the situations which come in our way and still maintaining health is not an easy task. But nothing is impossible, impossible is the word that itself says "I'm possible". After all we are human, we have feelings and emotions like happiness, sadness, anger and so on. Everyday we go through these emotions and sometimes we stress ourselves when limit is crossed.

Stress is definitely a cause of hypertension. Every one of us reacts differently to stress. Some of us smoke, take drink, cry, eat too much or less, etc. Because of stress, adrenaline hormone is released which cause vasoconstriction.

What actually is stress?

It's a strain which we take upon us due to the external or internal factors like:

o No money, no job. Today's big problem

o Job dissatisfaction,

o Spoilt relationship with superior.

o Not able to meet the time line.

o Social stress, pressure of society,

o Unmarried peoples get loneliness.

o Poverty.

Stress can be relieved by stress management. Everybody is blessed with some or the other skills, some people are good in painting, some are good in singing, dancing and some good in their colonial hand. Try the things which makes you feel relax. Other options are also there like:

o Meditation

o Yoga

o Sports

o Listening to music

o Reading

Everybody starting from children to old age population is fond of eating. How many of us can control over eating habits? Hardly any. We like French fries, pizzas, canned food but guess the content of sodium! Our daily requirement of sodium is 1500mg, less than a teaspoon. But two slices of pizza exceed our daily requirement. What happens next? Sodium imbalance, kidney failure, water retention, weight gain, edema, loss of potassium which all are reasons for hypertension.

We can overcome all of these especially by changing our lifestyle. Hypertension can be controlled by DASH (Dietary approaches to stop hypertension) plan and regular regime of workout and control over diet. Eating food containing high potassium like nuts, legumes and lowering sodium intake by avoiding especially canned or preserved food items.

Whenever we are happy we celebrate with a Champagne, which is a must. Social drinking doesn't impact on our body much. But addiction of alcohol drinking which goes hand in hand with smoking too, does impact. Not much is known about direct relationship between alcohol addiction and hypertension. But studies show that after alcohol consumption it sets on sympathetic activity and vasoconstriction related hormones are released and thus becomes a cause of hypertension.

Alcohol consumption coupled with other disorders like obesity could synergistically affect blood pressure.

Only way to overcome alcohol related hypertension is to quit dependency on alcohol and smoking. Hard to do but not impossible. Engage yourself with family members or some kind of sports or support group which does not remind of drinking and smoking.

These were the ways which we implement in our lives and get rid of hypertension. But to bring down the blood pressure ⬚uickly antihypertensive medicines are available. Some of them are as stated:

o Diuretics such as bumetanide, epitizide

o Vasodilators such as sodium nitroprusside

o Antagonist of adrenaline receptor like timolol, terazosin

Again there is a saying that ignorance is bliss, but in body science ignorance can be life threatening.

CHAPTER 5- A NUTRITIONAL

What is a Healthy High Blood Pressure Nutrition?

The Western World is today full of people suffering from the life threatening condition high blood pressure. To ensure good health is maintained it is vital that we strive to maintain healthy blood pressure and reduce elevated blood pressure. Diet is a major corner stone in this quest. There is a huge amount of medical evidence which supports the link between high blood pressure and diet. Perhaps however, linking a certain food with a specific medical problem is taking this a bit too literally.

It is well documented that a diet which incorporates lots of fresh fruit and vegetables, one which is typically followed by a vegetarian for example has great success in reducing blood pressure. A diet which includes a lot of fast food and contains a lot of saturated fat and salt is a disaster in terms of blood pressure. This on the face of it seems simple and straightforward, but it does not always follow. Many people who have followed the Atkins diet have also found a reduction in their blood pressure.

A nutritional Diet Guidelines

It is a well-known fact that heart diseases and excess body weight are related. Obesity, heavy alcohol consumption and lack of activity are the main factors causing high blood pressure. Too much body fat leads to an increased risk of health problems through clogging the blood vessels with cholesterol. That is why the successful treatment of high blood pressure starts with following a diet specifically aimed at reducing high blood pressure.

If you already have high blood pressure, you cannot reverse it to low permanently. Instead, you can control your high blood pressure by taking a prescribed medication and amending your diet. Research has shown that a high blood pressure diet can effectively prevent blood pressure from rising above normal.

Today, most of our meals still contain more fat than the government recommends, and most of the vending machines and fast-food options do not meet the nutritional standards set by the U.S. government. With fast-food snacks available at every corner, it's often hard to switch to a healthy diet.

High blood pressure diets are designed to decrease sodium, increase potassium, and lessen calories. This way you will maintain a reasonable weight. This diet consists of foods that are delicious and low in fat such as whole grains, fruits, vegetables, low-fat dairy products and lean proteins.

Here are some simple tips to help you follow your high blood pressure diet guidelines:

1. Make sure you eat a healthy breakfast. Eating in the morning will increase your energy and will help you avoid snacks before lunch. A □uick breakfast can be as easy as a bowl of cereal, a slice of whole-wheat toast, cereal bar or fresh fruit.

2. When following your high blood pressure diet, your daily food intake must include foods from five food groups:

- Protein: Eat meats that are lower in fat, such as chicken, turkey, tuna, or low-fat luncheon meats. Make salads with a low fat meat or vegetables and light salad dressing.

- Grains: Always try eating a whole wheat version of your favorite bread, be it a loaf, a bagel or a roll.

- Vegetables: Eat tomatoes, peppers, baby carrots and other colorful vegetables as many as you like. The brighter the vegetable, the more antioxidant vitamin A it contains.

- Fruits: Fruits should be eaten fresh. Fruit has fiber and healthy calories, and you will want to eat less during the day. Juice has fructose which fills up with energy. That's why juice should become a part of a healthy breakfast along with a cereal.

- Dairy: Try low-fat or non-fat milk, non-fat chocolate milk, and low-fat cheese. Basically, any type of cottage cheese or yogurt goes well with fruit.

If you want to avoid facing complicated and often life-threatening conse uences of high blood pressure, you may want to ensure that you and your family eat healthy meals that don't pack on the pounds and raise your cholesterol.

Emphasizing healthy food choices can help you enjoy your meals without excessive fat, sugar, and calories. Healthy food choices can be a carry-over from healthy menu and meal planning at home while managing your high blood pressure with diet.

Switching to a diet without excessive fat and salt and staying fit will help you loose weight and can help prevent or at least delay heart-related problems.

Along with monitoring and medication treatment, a high blood pressure diet can help control your blood pressure and reduce your risk of stroke, kidney and heart failure and heart attack.

So what constitutes a good high blood pressure diet?

The answer to this is simple, everything can be eaten in moderation. A mixed, well balanced diet is all that is re□uired. Salt for example is always haled as being extremely bad for you and should be avoided. The truth is that the body needs salt to function correctly. The excesses found in processed foods are detrimental as the balance of minerals in the body is disrupted these also include potassium and magnesium as well as sodium which is found in salt. In reasonable quantities salt can be included in the diet and the same can be said for lean cuts of meat and low fat dairy products.

Dietary Approaches to Stop Hypertension or DASH for short is an officially recommended diet for those who re□uire a high blood pressure diet. These types of "officially recommended" diets usually fill people with fear. In this instance the diet recommended is a sensible, well balanced diet which we would all do well to take heed of even if we do not suffer from high blood pressure.

The diet recommends plenty of freshly prepared fruit and vegetables with lean meat and low fat dairy products - a simple low fat, low sugar diet. What it promotes is a back to basics approach. Buying fresh produce and preparing simple healthy meals in your own kitchen replacing the processed ready meal diet.

The only problem with this diet as with most diets is that it lays down strict portion sizes and the number of servings which should be consumed in each food group. I think that a balanced diet is more about eating foods according to the cycle of nature i.e. foods which are in season and plentiful from local sources.

Ways to Reduce High BP

High blood pressure refers to the condition in which blood moves with a greater pressure in the arteries. Blood pressure is measured in a two numbers format such as 120/80. If the number is 140/95 or more, it is said to be high blood pressure. BP in between 120/80 and 140/95 is called pre-hypertension. There are no visible symptoms of high blood pressure but it can cause life threatening conditions. It is advised to go for a regular blood pressure check up after the age of 18 years to reduce the risk.

There are two types of high blood pressure conditions: high BP and pre-hypertension which can raise the risk of stroke, heart problems, kidney failure and heart attack. One should take a balanced diet and make some changes in the lifestyle to reduce the risk.

Some of the changes which can be made in lifestyle and diet for reducing the risk are given below. These are effective and safe methods.

Reduce intake sodium in diet: According to some research it has been found that increased intake of sodium in diet can increase the BP level in some people, although it is not true for all. Depending on the way the body reacts one can reduce intake sodium in diet. Sodium is found in high □uantity in most of the packaged and preserved food products. It is advised to take sodium amount less than 1500 mg in a day for people who belong to African American group and people who belong to other ethnics group but are old. Healthy people should take less than 2300 mg sodium in a day. High sodium is found in chips, canned vegetables, cheese, bread, soups and there are certain drugs which contain a good amount of sodium and one should be careful before taking such drugs.

Fresh vegetables and food products are generally low in salt and sodium is naturally found in certain food products such as meat, fruits, vegetables, grains and dairy products. One should reduce salt in food preparation and use more herbs. Smoked and cured dishes are mostly high in sodium and it should be avoided.

Avoid Tobacco and alcohol: Tobacco products can be very damaging to people who suffer from high blood pressure. As it raises heart beat and it can temporarily increase the blood pressure. It is advised to reduce intake of certain tobacco products to reduce the risk of heart attack. Alcohol can raise BP and one should not take it.

Adverse effect of obesity: One should try to maintain a good weight and do not get obese as it raises the risk.

Saturated and trans fats: Reduce intake of food products which are low in saturated fats and trans fat. A diet rich in fruits and vegetables should be taken.

Increase food products high in minerals: The diet should be low in cholesterol but high in certain minerals such as calcium, magnesium and potassium. The diet should be good in fibers. Intake of protein should be moderately high.

There are really no black and white answer to what a good high blood pressure diet is. All foods should be eaten in moderation in a varied, sensible diet - although processed food should be avoided! Following this simple advise could help reduce your weight and most importantly your blood pressure and possibly your grocery bill.

CHAPTER 6- MINDSET APPROACH

It is a common assumption that the stress of everyday living is directly related to hypertension. However, such is not the case. Amazingly, there is no definitive data that correlates chronic high blood pressure to the immediate impact of stress. In our fast paced modern world we are constantly confronted with stress situations such as traffic tie-ups, financial difficulties, demanding work loads and strained interpersonal relationships. It seems to make sense that constant exposure to such taxing circumstances causes high blood pressure. Though there is no evidence of a direct link between stress and hypertension it is generally accepted that minimizing stress contributes to better overall health.

The Fight or Flight Response: The human body is designed with a mechanism for self preservation commonly known as the Fight or Flight Response. When we encounter a perceived threat our bodies react with a surge in cortisol and adrenalin. These hormones ready the body to either face the threat head on or make a hasty retreat. This reaction was essential in more primitive times when physical danger was more common. However, the body makes no distinction between an actual threat and a perceived one. These hormones are released in either case but if we do not take either action our bodies are left with elevated levels of both hormones. Unfortunately, there will be a rise in blood pressure until these levels eventually drop back to normal levels.

There is no substantive data indicating a cause and effect relationship between stress and high blood pressure. However there is some conjecture among researchers that there may be an indirect link between the two. However, negative lifestyle habits such as tobacco use, alcohol consumption, bad dietary habits and poor sleep hygiene are more closely associated with stress and therefore indirectly implicated with hypertension. There is an additional consideration that the emotional stress experienced by sufferers of panic disorder or chronic anxiety may cause non-compliance with their hypertension medication regimen. Conse□uently, it becomes evident that stress reduction has major health benefits.

Managing Stress

Stress seems and unavoidable fact of life today. Though there may be little we can do to eliminate the actual causes of stress in our lives there are some techni□ues we can employ to help us cope.

Putting Things Into Perspective

It is important to make the distinction between an actual physical threat and mental stress. While not minimizing the significance of everyday stress we must learn that the majority of them are not real physical threats. This will allow us to adjust our mindset from fear to mental preparedness.

Con□uering Stress

There are several popular techni□ues which are effective in lowering the body's reaction to stress. Some of these include progressive relaxation, meditation, yoga, physical exercise and a proper sleep schedule. Avoid undue worrying about your hypertension. It is possible to be attentive regarding your blood pressure without falling into a downward spiral of worry and further stress.

Your mental attitude has a significant impact on your ability to manage your hypertension. A proactive approach which incorporates a combination of medication, lifestyle changes and stress management techniques will provide you with a sense of empowerment. Bringing stress under control both physically and mentally will bring your blood pressure under control as well.

CONCLUSION

See your doctor for checkups or tests as often as he or she recommends. Your treatment plan as prescribed by your doctor may change over time, and regular checkups allow you and your doctor to know whether your blood pressure is rising so that your treatment plan can be Quickly altered as necessary. During checkups, you can ask your doctor or health care team any Questions you have about your lifestyle or medicine treatments.

Keeping track of your blood pressure is vital. Have your blood pressure checked on the schedule your doctor advises. You may want to learn how to check your blood pressure at home. Your doctor can help you with this. Each time you check your own blood pressure, you should write down your numbers and the date

REFERENCE

* Williams B, Poulter NR, Brown MJ, et al. Guidelines for management of hypertension: report of the fourth working party of the British Hypertension Society, 2004- BHS IV. J Hum Hypertens.

* Whitworth JA. World Health Organisation, International Society of Hypertension Writing Group. 2003 World Health Organization (WHO)/International Society of Hypertension (ISH) statement on management of hypertension.

* Erdine S, Ari O, Zanchetti A, et al. ESH-ESC guidelines for the management of hypertension.

* Appel LJ, American Society of Hypertension Writing Group. Giles TD, et al. ASH Position Paper: dietary approaches to lower blood pressure.

* Appel LJ, Brands MW, Daniels SR, et al. Dietary approaches to prevent and treat hypertension: a scientific statement from the American Heart Association.

* Chobanian AV, Bakris GL, Black HR, et al. The Seventh Report of the Joint National Committee on Prevention,

Detection, Evaluation, and Treatment of High Blood Pressure:

* Cook NR, Cohen J, Hebert PR, et al. Implications of small reductions in diastolic blood pressure for primary prevention. Arch Intern Med.

* Chen ST, Maruthur NM, Appel LJ. The effect of dietary patterns on estimated coronary heart disease risk: results from the Dietary Approaches to Stop Hypertension (DASH) trial. Circ Cardiovasc Qual Outcomes.

* Craddick SR, Elmer PJ, Obarzanek E, et al. The DASH diet and blood pressure.

* Swain JF, McCarron PB, Hamilton EF, et al. Characteristics of the diet patterns tested in the optimal macronutrient intake trial to prevent heart disease (OMNIHeart): options for a heart-healthy diet.

* Miller ER, 3rd, Erlinger TP, Appel LJ. The effects of macronutrients on blood pressure and lipids: an overview of the DASH and OMNIHeart trials.

* Appel LJ, Champagne CM, Harsha DW, et al. Effects of comprehensive lifestyle modification on blood pressure control: main results of the PREMIER clinical trial. JAMA.

* Mahtani KR. Simple advice to reduce salt intake. Br J Gen Pract. 2009;59(567):786–787.

* Pérez-López FR, Chedraui P, Haya J, Cuadros JL. Effects of the Mediterranean diet on longevity and age-related morbid conditions.